Personal Data

Name _____

Phone _____

Address _____

MW00892396

Incase of Emergency, Please Contact

Name _____

Phone _____

Address _____

Essential Contacts

Doctor _____

Pharmacy _____

Eye Clinic _____

Dentist _____

Name	*Name*
Cell:	Cell:
Work:	Work:
Home:	Home:
Email:	Email:
Other:	Other:

Name	*Name*
Cell:	Cell:
Work:	Work:
Home:	Home:
Email:	Email:
Other:	Other:

Note

Note

Note

Week				Weight

Date	Meal	Before	After	Note
MONDAY ___/___/___	Breakfast			
	Lunch			
	Dinner			
	Bedtime			
TUESDAY ___/___/___	Breakfast			
	Lunch			
	Dinner			
	Bedtime			
WEDNESDAY ___/___/___	Breakfast			
	Lunch			
	Dinner			
	Bedtime			
THURSDAY ___/___/___	Breakfast			
	Lunch			
	Dinner			
	Bedtime			
FRIDAY ___/___/___	Breakfast			
	Lunch			
	Dinner			
	Bedtime			
SATURDAY ___/___/___	Breakfast			
	Lunch			
	Dinner			
	Bedtime			
SUNDAY ___/___/___	Breakfast			
	Lunch			
	Dinner			
	Bedtime			

NOTE

Week				Weight

Date	Meal	Before	After	Note
MONDAY __/__/__	Breakfast			
	Lunch			
	Dinner			
	Bedtime			
TUESDAY __/__/__	Breakfast			
	Lunch			
	Dinner			
	Bedtime			
WEDNESDAY __/__/__	Breakfast			
	Lunch			
	Dinner			
	Bedtime			
THURSDAY __/__/__	Breakfast			
	Lunch			
	Dinner			
	Bedtime			
FRIDAY __/__/__	Breakfast			
	Lunch			
	Dinner			
	Bedtime			
SATURDAY __/__/__	Breakfast			
	Lunch			
	Dinner			
	Bedtime			
SUNDAY __/__/__	Breakfast			
	Lunch			
	Dinner			
	Bedtime			

NOTE

Week				Weight

Date	Meal	Before	After	Note
MONDAY ___/___/___	Breakfast			
	Lunch			
	Dinner			
	Bedtime			
TUESDAY ___/___/___	Breakfast			
	Lunch			
	Dinner			
	Bedtime			
WEDNESDAY ___/___/___	Breakfast			
	Lunch			
	Dinner			
	Bedtime			
THURSDAY ___/___/___	Breakfast			
	Lunch			
	Dinner			
	Bedtime			
FRIDAY ___/___/___	Breakfast			
	Lunch			
	Dinner			
	Bedtime			
SATURDAY ___/___/___	Breakfast			
	Lunch			
	Dinner			
	Bedtime			
SUNDAY ___/___/___	Breakfast			
	Lunch			
	Dinner			
	Bedtime			

NOTE

Week					Weight

Date	Meal	Before	After	Note
MONDAY __/__/__	Breakfast			
	Lunch			
	Dinner			
	Bedtime			
TUESDAY __/__/__	Breakfast			
	Lunch			
	Dinner			
	Bedtime			
WEDNESDAY __/__/__	Breakfast			
	Lunch			
	Dinner			
	Bedtime			
THURSDAY __/__/__	Breakfast			
	Lunch			
	Dinner			
	Bedtime			
FRIDAY __/__/__	Breakfast			
	Lunch			
	Dinner			
	Bedtime			
SATURDAY __/__/__	Breakfast			
	Lunch			
	Dinner			
	Bedtime			
SUNDAY __/__/__	Breakfast			
	Lunch			
	Dinner			
	Bedtime			

NOTE

Week				Weight

Date	Meal	Before	After	Note
MONDAY ___/___/___	Breakfast			
	Lunch			
	Dinner			
	Bedtime			
TUESDAY ___/___/___	Breakfast			
	Lunch			
	Dinner			
	Bedtime			
WEDNESDAY ___/___/___	Breakfast			
	Lunch			
	Dinner			
	Bedtime			
THURSDAY ___/___/___	Breakfast			
	Lunch			
	Dinner			
	Bedtime			
FRIDAY ___/___/___	Breakfast			
	Lunch			
	Dinner			
	Bedtime			
SATURDAY ___/___/___	Breakfast			
	Lunch			
	Dinner			
	Bedtime			
SUNDAY ___/___/___	Breakfast			
	Lunch			
	Dinner			
	Bedtime			

NOTE

Week				Weight

Date	Meal	Before	After	Note
MONDAY __/__/__	Breakfast			
	Lunch			
	Dinner			
	Bedtime			
TUESDAY __/__/__	Breakfast			
	Lunch			
	Dinner			
	Bedtime			
WEDNESDAY __/__/__	Breakfast			
	Lunch			
	Dinner			
	Bedtime			
THURSDAY __/__/__	Breakfast			
	Lunch			
	Dinner			
	Bedtime			
FRIDAY __/__/__	Breakfast			
	Lunch			
	Dinner			
	Bedtime			
SATURDAY __/__/__	Breakfast			
	Lunch			
	Dinner			
	Bedtime			
SUNDAY __/__/__	Breakfast			
	Lunch			
	Dinner			
	Bedtime			

NOTE

Week				Weight

Date	Meal	Before	After	Note
MONDAY ___/___/___	Breakfast			
	Lunch			
	Dinner			
	Bedtime			
TUESDAY ___/___/___	Breakfast			
	Lunch			
	Dinner			
	Bedtime			
WEDNESDAY ___/___/___	Breakfast			
	Lunch			
	Dinner			
	Bedtime			
THURSDAY ___/___/___	Breakfast			
	Lunch			
	Dinner			
	Bedtime			
FRIDAY ___/___/___	Breakfast			
	Lunch			
	Dinner			
	Bedtime			
SATURDAY ___/___/___	Breakfast			
	Lunch			
	Dinner			
	Bedtime			
SUNDAY ___/___/___	Breakfast			
	Lunch			
	Dinner			
	Bedtime			

NOTE

Week				Weight

Date	Meal	Before	After	Note
MONDAY ___/___/___	Breakfast			
	Lunch			
	Dinner			
	Bedtime			
TUESDAY ___/___/___	Breakfast			
	Lunch			
	Dinner			
	Bedtime			
WEDNESDAY ___/___/___	Breakfast			
	Lunch			
	Dinner			
	Bedtime			
THURSDAY ___/___/___	Breakfast			
	Lunch			
	Dinner			
	Bedtime			
FRIDAY ___/___/___	Breakfast			
	Lunch			
	Dinner			
	Bedtime			
SATURDAY ___/___/___	Breakfast			
	Lunch			
	Dinner			
	Bedtime			
SUNDAY ___/___/___	Breakfast			
	Lunch			
	Dinner			
	Bedtime			

NOTE

Week				Weight

Date	Meal	Before	After	Note
MONDAY ___/___/___	Breakfast			
	Lunch			
	Dinner			
	Bedtime			
TUESDAY ___/___/___	Breakfast			
	Lunch			
	Dinner			
	Bedtime			
WEDNESDAY ___/___/___	Breakfast			
	Lunch			
	Dinner			
	Bedtime			
THURSDAY ___/___/___	Breakfast			
	Lunch			
	Dinner			
	Bedtime			
FRIDAY ___/___/___	Breakfast			
	Lunch			
	Dinner			
	Bedtime			
SATURDAY ___/___/___	Breakfast			
	Lunch			
	Dinner			
	Bedtime			
SUNDAY ___/___/___	Breakfast			
	Lunch			
	Dinner			
	Bedtime			

NOTE

Week				Weight

Date	Meal	Before	After	Note
MONDAY ___/___/___	Breakfast			
	Lunch			
	Dinner			
	Bedtime			
TUESDAY ___/___/___	Breakfast			
	Lunch			
	Dinner			
	Bedtime			
WEDNESDAY ___/___/___	Breakfast			
	Lunch			
	Dinner			
	Bedtime			
THURSDAY ___/___/___	Breakfast			
	Lunch			
	Dinner			
	Bedtime			
FRIDAY ___/___/___	Breakfast			
	Lunch			
	Dinner			
	Bedtime			
SATURDAY ___/___/___	Breakfast			
	Lunch			
	Dinner			
	Bedtime			
SUNDAY ___/___/___	Breakfast			
	Lunch			
	Dinner			
	Bedtime			

NOTE

Week				Weight

Date	Meal	Before	After	Note
MONDAY ___/___/___	Breakfast			
	Lunch			
	Dinner			
	Bedtime			
TUESDAY ___/___/___	Breakfast			
	Lunch			
	Dinner			
	Bedtime			
WEDNESDAY ___/___/___	Breakfast			
	Lunch			
	Dinner			
	Bedtime			
THURSDAY ___/___/___	Breakfast			
	Lunch			
	Dinner			
	Bedtime			
FRIDAY ___/___/___	Breakfast			
	Lunch			
	Dinner			
	Bedtime			
SATURDAY ___/___/___	Breakfast			
	Lunch			
	Dinner			
	Bedtime			
SUNDAY ___/___/___	Breakfast			
	Lunch			
	Dinner			
	Bedtime			

NOTE

Week				Weight

Date	Meal	Before	After	Note
MONDAY ___/___/___	Breakfast			
	Lunch			
	Dinner			
	Bedtime			
TUESDAY ___/___/___	Breakfast			
	Lunch			
	Dinner			
	Bedtime			
WEDNESDAY ___/___/___	Breakfast			
	Lunch			
	Dinner			
	Bedtime			
THURSDAY ___/___/___	Breakfast			
	Lunch			
	Dinner			
	Bedtime			
FRIDAY ___/___/___	Breakfast			
	Lunch			
	Dinner			
	Bedtime			
SATURDAY ___/___/___	Breakfast			
	Lunch			
	Dinner			
	Bedtime			
SUNDAY ___/___/___	Breakfast			
	Lunch			
	Dinner			
	Bedtime			

NOTE _____

Week				Weight

Date	Meal	Before	After	Note
MONDAY ___/___/___	Breakfast			
	Lunch			
	Dinner			
	Bedtime			
TUESDAY ___/___/___	Breakfast			
	Lunch			
	Dinner			
	Bedtime			
WEDNESDAY ___/___/___	Breakfast			
	Lunch			
	Dinner			
	Bedtime			
THURSDAY ___/___/___	Breakfast			
	Lunch			
	Dinner			
	Bedtime			
FRIDAY ___/___/___	Breakfast			
	Lunch			
	Dinner			
	Bedtime			
SATURDAY ___/___/___	Breakfast			
	Lunch			
	Dinner			
	Bedtime			
SUNDAY ___/___/___	Breakfast			
	Lunch			
	Dinner			
	Bedtime			

NOTE

Week				Weight

Date	Meal	Before	After	Note
MONDAY ___/___/___	Breakfast			
	Lunch			
	Dinner			
	Bedtime			
TUESDAY ___/___/___	Breakfast			
	Lunch			
	Dinner			
	Bedtime			
WEDNESDAY ___/___/___	Breakfast			
	Lunch			
	Dinner			
	Bedtime			
THURSDAY ___/___/___	Breakfast			
	Lunch			
	Dinner			
	Bedtime			
FRIDAY ___/___/___	Breakfast			
	Lunch			
	Dinner			
	Bedtime			
SATURDAY ___/___/___	Breakfast			
	Lunch			
	Dinner			
	Bedtime			
SUNDAY ___/___/___	Breakfast			
	Lunch			
	Dinner			
	Bedtime			

NOTE

Week				Weight

Date	Meal	Before	After	Note
MONDAY ___/___/___	Breakfast			
	Lunch			
	Dinner			
	Bedtime			
TUESDAY ___/___/___	Breakfast			
	Lunch			
	Dinner			
	Bedtime			
WEDNESDAY ___/___/___	Breakfast			
	Lunch			
	Dinner			
	Bedtime			
THURSDAY ___/___/___	Breakfast			
	Lunch			
	Dinner			
	Bedtime			
FRIDAY ___/___/___	Breakfast			
	Lunch			
	Dinner			
	Bedtime			
SATURDAY ___/___/___	Breakfast			
	Lunch			
	Dinner			
	Bedtime			
SUNDAY ___/___/___	Breakfast			
	Lunch			
	Dinner			
	Bedtime			

NOTE

Week				Weight

Date	Meal	Before	After	Note
MONDAY __/__/__	Breakfast			
	Lunch			
	Dinner			
	Bedtime			
TUESDAY __/__/__	Breakfast			
	Lunch			
	Dinner			
	Bedtime			
WEDNESDAY __/__/__	Breakfast			
	Lunch			
	Dinner			
	Bedtime			
THURSDAY __/__/__	Breakfast			
	Lunch			
	Dinner			
	Bedtime			
FRIDAY __/__/__	Breakfast			
	Lunch			
	Dinner			
	Bedtime			
SATURDAY __/__/__	Breakfast			
	Lunch			
	Dinner			
	Bedtime			
SUNDAY __/__/__	Breakfast			
	Lunch			
	Dinner			
	Bedtime			

NOTE

Week				Weight

Date	Meal	Before	After	Note
MONDAY ___/___/___	Breakfast			
	Lunch			
	Dinner			
	Bedtime			
TUESDAY ___/___/___	Breakfast			
	Lunch			
	Dinner			
	Bedtime			
WEDNESDAY ___/___/___	Breakfast			
	Lunch			
	Dinner			
	Bedtime			
THURSDAY ___/___/___	Breakfast			
	Lunch			
	Dinner			
	Bedtime			
FRIDAY ___/___/___	Breakfast			
	Lunch			
	Dinner			
	Bedtime			
SATURDAY ___/___/___	Breakfast			
	Lunch			
	Dinner			
	Bedtime			
SUNDAY ___/___/___	Breakfast			
	Lunch			
	Dinner			
	Bedtime			

NOTE

Week				Weight

Date	Meal	Before	After	Note
MONDAY __/__/__	Breakfast			
	Lunch			
	Dinner			
	Bedtime			
TUESDAY __/__/__	Breakfast			
	Lunch			
	Dinner			
	Bedtime			
WEDNESDAY __/__/__	Breakfast			
	Lunch			
	Dinner			
	Bedtime			
THURSDAY __/__/__	Breakfast			
	Lunch			
	Dinner			
	Bedtime			
FRIDAY __/__/__	Breakfast			
	Lunch			
	Dinner			
	Bedtime			
SATURDAY __/__/__	Breakfast			
	Lunch			
	Dinner			
	Bedtime			
SUNDAY __/__/__	Breakfast			
	Lunch			
	Dinner			
	Bedtime			

NOTE

Week				Weight

Date	Meal	Before	After	Note
MONDAY ___/___/___	Breakfast			
	Lunch			
	Dinner			
	Bedtime			
TUESDAY ___/___/___	Breakfast			
	Lunch			
	Dinner			
	Bedtime			
WEDNESDAY ___/___/___	Breakfast			
	Lunch			
	Dinner			
	Bedtime			
THURSDAY ___/___/___	Breakfast			
	Lunch			
	Dinner			
	Bedtime			
FRIDAY ___/___/___	Breakfast			
	Lunch			
	Dinner			
	Bedtime			
SATURDAY ___/___/___	Breakfast			
	Lunch			
	Dinner			
	Bedtime			
SUNDAY ___/___/___	Breakfast			
	Lunch			
	Dinner			
	Bedtime			

NOTE

Week				Weight

Date	Meal	Before	After	Note
MONDAY __/__/__	Breakfast			
	Lunch			
	Dinner			
	Bedtime			
TUESDAY __/__/__	Breakfast			
	Lunch			
	Dinner			
	Bedtime			
WEDNESDAY __/__/__	Breakfast			
	Lunch			
	Dinner			
	Bedtime			
THURSDAY __/__/__	Breakfast			
	Lunch			
	Dinner			
	Bedtime			
FRIDAY __/__/__	Breakfast			
	Lunch			
	Dinner			
	Bedtime			
SATURDAY __/__/__	Breakfast			
	Lunch			
	Dinner			
	Bedtime			
SUNDAY __/__/__	Breakfast			
	Lunch			
	Dinner			
	Bedtime			

NOTE

Week				Weight

Date	Meal	Before	After	Note
MONDAY ___/___/___	Breakfast			
	Lunch			
	Dinner			
	Bedtime			
TUESDAY ___/___/___	Breakfast			
	Lunch			
	Dinner			
	Bedtime			
WEDNESDAY ___/___/___	Breakfast			
	Lunch			
	Dinner			
	Bedtime			
THURSDAY ___/___/___	Breakfast			
	Lunch			
	Dinner			
	Bedtime			
FRIDAY ___/___/___	Breakfast			
	Lunch			
	Dinner			
	Bedtime			
SATURDAY ___/___/___	Breakfast			
	Lunch			
	Dinner			
	Bedtime			
SUNDAY ___/___/___	Breakfast			
	Lunch			
	Dinner			
	Bedtime			

NOTE

Week				Weight

Date	Meal	Before	After	Note
MONDAY __/__/__	Breakfast			
	Lunch			
	Dinner			
	Bedtime			
TUESDAY __/__/__	Breakfast			
	Lunch			
	Dinner			
	Bedtime			
WEDNESDAY __/__/__	Breakfast			
	Lunch			
	Dinner			
	Bedtime			
THURSDAY __/__/__	Breakfast			
	Lunch			
	Dinner			
	Bedtime			
FRIDAY __/__/__	Breakfast			
	Lunch			
	Dinner			
	Bedtime			
SATURDAY __/__/__	Breakfast			
	Lunch			
	Dinner			
	Bedtime			
SUNDAY __/__/__	Breakfast			
	Lunch			
	Dinner			
	Bedtime			

NOTE

Week				Weight

Date	Meal	Before	After	Note
MONDAY __/__/__	Breakfast			
	Lunch			
	Dinner			
	Bedtime			
TUESDAY __/__/__	Breakfast			
	Lunch			
	Dinner			
	Bedtime			
WEDNESDAY __/__/__	Breakfast			
	Lunch			
	Dinner			
	Bedtime			
THURSDAY __/__/__	Breakfast			
	Lunch			
	Dinner			
	Bedtime			
FRIDAY __/__/__	Breakfast			
	Lunch			
	Dinner			
	Bedtime			
SATURDAY __/__/__	Breakfast			
	Lunch			
	Dinner			
	Bedtime			
SUNDAY __/__/__	Breakfast			
	Lunch			
	Dinner			
	Bedtime			

NOTE

Week				Weight

Date	Meal	Before	After	Note
MONDAY __/__/__	Breakfast			
	Lunch			
	Dinner			
	Bedtime			
TUESDAY __/__/__	Breakfast			
	Lunch			
	Dinner			
	Bedtime			
WEDNESDAY __/__/__	Breakfast			
	Lunch			
	Dinner			
	Bedtime			
THURSDAY __/__/__	Breakfast			
	Lunch			
	Dinner			
	Bedtime			
FRIDAY __/__/__	Breakfast			
	Lunch			
	Dinner			
	Bedtime			
SATURDAY __/__/__	Breakfast			
	Lunch			
	Dinner			
	Bedtime			
SUNDAY __/__/__	Breakfast			
	Lunch			
	Dinner			
	Bedtime			

NOTE

Week				Weight

Date	Meal	Before	After	Note
MONDAY __/__/__	Breakfast			
	Lunch			
	Dinner			
	Bedtime			
TUESDAY __/__/__	Breakfast			
	Lunch			
	Dinner			
	Bedtime			
WEDNESDAY __/__/__	Breakfast			
	Lunch			
	Dinner			
	Bedtime			
THURSDAY __/__/__	Breakfast			
	Lunch			
	Dinner			
	Bedtime			
FRIDAY __/__/__	Breakfast			
	Lunch			
	Dinner			
	Bedtime			
SATURDAY __/__/__	Breakfast			
	Lunch			
	Dinner			
	Bedtime			
SUNDAY __/__/__	Breakfast			
	Lunch			
	Dinner			
	Bedtime			

NOTE

Week				Weight

Date	Meal	Before	After	Note
MONDAY ___/___/___	Breakfast			
	Lunch			
	Dinner			
	Bedtime			
TUESDAY ___/___/___	Breakfast			
	Lunch			
	Dinner			
	Bedtime			
WEDNESDAY ___/___/___	Breakfast			
	Lunch			
	Dinner			
	Bedtime			
THURSDAY ___/___/___	Breakfast			
	Lunch			
	Dinner			
	Bedtime			
FRIDAY ___/___/___	Breakfast			
	Lunch			
	Dinner			
	Bedtime			
SATURDAY ___/___/___	Breakfast			
	Lunch			
	Dinner			
	Bedtime			
SUNDAY ___/___/___	Breakfast			
	Lunch			
	Dinner			
	Bedtime			

NOTE

Week				Weight

Date	Meal	Before	After	Note
MONDAY ___/___/___	Breakfast			
	Lunch			
	Dinner			
	Bedtime			
TUESDAY ___/___/___	Breakfast			
	Lunch			
	Dinner			
	Bedtime			
WEDNESDAY ___/___/___	Breakfast			
	Lunch			
	Dinner			
	Bedtime			
THURSDAY ___/___/___	Breakfast			
	Lunch			
	Dinner			
	Bedtime			
FRIDAY ___/___/___	Breakfast			
	Lunch			
	Dinner			
	Bedtime			
SATURDAY ___/___/___	Breakfast			
	Lunch			
	Dinner			
	Bedtime			
SUNDAY ___/___/___	Breakfast			
	Lunch			
	Dinner			
	Bedtime			

NOTE

Week				Weight

Date	Meal	Before	After	Note
MONDAY ___/___/___	Breakfast			
	Lunch			
	Dinner			
	Bedtime			
TUESDAY ___/___/___	Breakfast			
	Lunch			
	Dinner			
	Bedtime			
WEDNESDAY ___/___/___	Breakfast			
	Lunch			
	Dinner			
	Bedtime			
THURSDAY ___/___/___	Breakfast			
	Lunch			
	Dinner			
	Bedtime			
FRIDAY ___/___/___	Breakfast			
	Lunch			
	Dinner			
	Bedtime			
SATURDAY ___/___/___	Breakfast			
	Lunch			
	Dinner			
	Bedtime			
SUNDAY ___/___/___	Breakfast			
	Lunch			
	Dinner			
	Bedtime			

NOTE

Week		Weight		

Date	Meal	Before	After	Note
MONDAY ___/___/___	Breakfast			
	Lunch			
	Dinner			
	Bedtime			
TUESDAY ___/___/___	Breakfast			
	Lunch			
	Dinner			
	Bedtime			
WEDNESDAY ___/___/___	Breakfast			
	Lunch			
	Dinner			
	Bedtime			
THURSDAY ___/___/___	Breakfast			
	Lunch			
	Dinner			
	Bedtime			
FRIDAY ___/___/___	Breakfast			
	Lunch			
	Dinner			
	Bedtime			
SATURDAY ___/___/___	Breakfast			
	Lunch			
	Dinner			
	Bedtime			
SUNDAY ___/___/___	Breakfast			
	Lunch			
	Dinner			
	Bedtime			

NOTE

Week				Weight

Date	Meal	Before	After	Note
MONDAY __/__/__	Breakfast			
	Lunch			
	Dinner			
	Bedtime			
TUESDAY __/__/__	Breakfast			
	Lunch			
	Dinner			
	Bedtime			
WEDNESDAY __/__/__	Breakfast			
	Lunch			
	Dinner			
	Bedtime			
THURSDAY __/__/__	Breakfast			
	Lunch			
	Dinner			
	Bedtime			
FRIDAY __/__/__	Breakfast			
	Lunch			
	Dinner			
	Bedtime			
SATURDAY __/__/__	Breakfast			
	Lunch			
	Dinner			
	Bedtime			
SUNDAY __/__/__	Breakfast			
	Lunch			
	Dinner			
	Bedtime			

NOTE

Week				Weight

Date	Meal	Before	After	Note
MONDAY ___/___/___	Breakfast			
	Lunch			
	Dinner			
	Bedtime			
TUESDAY ___/___/___	Breakfast			
	Lunch			
	Dinner			
	Bedtime			
WEDNESDAY ___/___/___	Breakfast			
	Lunch			
	Dinner			
	Bedtime			
THURSDAY ___/___/___	Breakfast			
	Lunch			
	Dinner			
	Bedtime			
FRIDAY ___/___/___	Breakfast			
	Lunch			
	Dinner			
	Bedtime			
SATURDAY ___/___/___	Breakfast			
	Lunch			
	Dinner			
	Bedtime			
SUNDAY ___/___/___	Breakfast			
	Lunch			
	Dinner			
	Bedtime			

NOTE

Week				Weight

Date	Meal	Before	After	Note
MONDAY __/__/__	Breakfast			
	Lunch			
	Dinner			
	Bedtime			
TUESDAY __/__/__	Breakfast			
	Lunch			
	Dinner			
	Bedtime			
WEDNESDAY __/__/__	Breakfast			
	Lunch			
	Dinner			
	Bedtime			
THURSDAY __/__/__	Breakfast			
	Lunch			
	Dinner			
	Bedtime			
FRIDAY __/__/__	Breakfast			
	Lunch			
	Dinner			
	Bedtime			
SATURDAY __/__/__	Breakfast			
	Lunch			
	Dinner			
	Bedtime			
SUNDAY __/__/__	Breakfast			
	Lunch			
	Dinner			
	Bedtime			

NOTE

| Week | | | | | | Weight | |

Date	Meal	Before	After	Note
MONDAY ___/___/___	Breakfast			
	Lunch			
	Dinner			
	Bedtime			
TUESDAY ___/___/___	Breakfast			
	Lunch			
	Dinner			
	Bedtime			
WEDNESDAY ___/___/___	Breakfast			
	Lunch			
	Dinner			
	Bedtime			
THURSDAY ___/___/___	Breakfast			
	Lunch			
	Dinner			
	Bedtime			
FRIDAY ___/___/___	Breakfast			
	Lunch			
	Dinner			
	Bedtime			
SATURDAY ___/___/___	Breakfast			
	Lunch			
	Dinner			
	Bedtime			
SUNDAY ___/___/___	Breakfast			
	Lunch			
	Dinner			
	Bedtime			

NOTE

Week				Weight

Date	Meal	Before	After	Note
MONDAY ___/___/___	Breakfast			
	Lunch			
	Dinner			
	Bedtime			
TUESDAY ___/___/___	Breakfast			
	Lunch			
	Dinner			
	Bedtime			
WEDNESDAY ___/___/___	Breakfast			
	Lunch			
	Dinner			
	Bedtime			
THURSDAY ___/___/___	Breakfast			
	Lunch			
	Dinner			
	Bedtime			
FRIDAY ___/___/___	Breakfast			
	Lunch			
	Dinner			
	Bedtime			
SATURDAY ___/___/___	Breakfast			
	Lunch			
	Dinner			
	Bedtime			
SUNDAY ___/___/___	Breakfast			
	Lunch			
	Dinner			
	Bedtime			

NOTE

Week				Weight

Date	Meal	Before	After	Note
MONDAY ___/___/___	Breakfast			
	Lunch			
	Dinner			
	Bedtime			
TUESDAY ___/___/___	Breakfast			
	Lunch			
	Dinner			
	Bedtime			
WEDNESDAY ___/___/___	Breakfast			
	Lunch			
	Dinner			
	Bedtime			
THURSDAY ___/___/___	Breakfast			
	Lunch			
	Dinner			
	Bedtime			
FRIDAY ___/___/___	Breakfast			
	Lunch			
	Dinner			
	Bedtime			
SATURDAY ___/___/___	Breakfast			
	Lunch			
	Dinner			
	Bedtime			
SUNDAY ___/___/___	Breakfast			
	Lunch			
	Dinner			
	Bedtime			

NOTE

Week				Weight

Date	Meal	Before	After	Note
MONDAY __/__/__	Breakfast			
	Lunch			
	Dinner			
	Bedtime			
TUESDAY __/__/__	Breakfast			
	Lunch			
	Dinner			
	Bedtime			
WEDNESDAY __/__/__	Breakfast			
	Lunch			
	Dinner			
	Bedtime			
THURSDAY __/__/__	Breakfast			
	Lunch			
	Dinner			
	Bedtime			
FRIDAY __/__/__	Breakfast			
	Lunch			
	Dinner			
	Bedtime			
SATURDAY __/__/__	Breakfast			
	Lunch			
	Dinner			
	Bedtime			
SUNDAY __/__/__	Breakfast			
	Lunch			
	Dinner			
	Bedtime			

NOTE

Week				Weight

Date	Meal	Before	After	Note
MONDAY ___/___/___	Breakfast			
	Lunch			
	Dinner			
	Bedtime			
TUESDAY ___/___/___	Breakfast			
	Lunch			
	Dinner			
	Bedtime			
WEDNESDAY ___/___/___	Breakfast			
	Lunch			
	Dinner			
	Bedtime			
THURSDAY ___/___/___	Breakfast			
	Lunch			
	Dinner			
	Bedtime			
FRIDAY ___/___/___	Breakfast			
	Lunch			
	Dinner			
	Bedtime			
SATURDAY ___/___/___	Breakfast			
	Lunch			
	Dinner			
	Bedtime			
SUNDAY ___/___/___	Breakfast			
	Lunch			
	Dinner			
	Bedtime			

NOTE

Week				Weight

Date	Meal	Before	After	Note
MONDAY ___/___/___	Breakfast			
	Lunch			
	Dinner			
	Bedtime			
TUESDAY ___/___/___	Breakfast			
	Lunch			
	Dinner			
	Bedtime			
WEDNESDAY ___/___/___	Breakfast			
	Lunch			
	Dinner			
	Bedtime			
THURSDAY ___/___/___	Breakfast			
	Lunch			
	Dinner			
	Bedtime			
FRIDAY ___/___/___	Breakfast			
	Lunch			
	Dinner			
	Bedtime			
SATURDAY ___/___/___	Breakfast			
	Lunch			
	Dinner			
	Bedtime			
SUNDAY ___/___/___	Breakfast			
	Lunch			
	Dinner			
	Bedtime			

NOTE

Week				Weight

Date	Meal	Before	After	Note
MONDAY ___/___/___	Breakfast			
	Lunch			
	Dinner			
	Bedtime			
TUESDAY ___/___/___	Breakfast			
	Lunch			
	Dinner			
	Bedtime			
WEDNESDAY ___/___/___	Breakfast			
	Lunch			
	Dinner			
	Bedtime			
THURSDAY ___/___/___	Breakfast			
	Lunch			
	Dinner			
	Bedtime			
FRIDAY ___/___/___	Breakfast			
	Lunch			
	Dinner			
	Bedtime			
SATURDAY ___/___/___	Breakfast			
	Lunch			
	Dinner			
	Bedtime			
SUNDAY ___/___/___	Breakfast			
	Lunch			
	Dinner			
	Bedtime			

NOTE

Week				Weight

Date	Meal	Before	After	Note
MONDAY __/__/__	Breakfast			
	Lunch			
	Dinner			
	Bedtime			
TUESDAY __/__/__	Breakfast			
	Lunch			
	Dinner			
	Bedtime			
WEDNESDAY __/__/__	Breakfast			
	Lunch			
	Dinner			
	Bedtime			
THURSDAY __/__/__	Breakfast			
	Lunch			
	Dinner			
	Bedtime			
FRIDAY __/__/__	Breakfast			
	Lunch			
	Dinner			
	Bedtime			
SATURDAY __/__/__	Breakfast			
	Lunch			
	Dinner			
	Bedtime			
SUNDAY __/__/__	Breakfast			
	Lunch			
	Dinner			
	Bedtime			

NOTE

Week				Weight

Date	Meal	Before	After	Note
MONDAY ___/___/___	Breakfast			
	Lunch			
	Dinner			
	Bedtime			
TUESDAY ___/___/___	Breakfast			
	Lunch			
	Dinner			
	Bedtime			
WEDNESDAY ___/___/___	Breakfast			
	Lunch			
	Dinner			
	Bedtime			
THURSDAY ___/___/___	Breakfast			
	Lunch			
	Dinner			
	Bedtime			
FRIDAY ___/___/___	Breakfast			
	Lunch			
	Dinner			
	Bedtime			
SATURDAY ___/___/___	Breakfast			
	Lunch			
	Dinner			
	Bedtime			
SUNDAY ___/___/___	Breakfast			
	Lunch			
	Dinner			
	Bedtime			

NOTE

Week				Weight

Date	Meal	Before	After	Note
MONDAY __/__/__	Breakfast			
	Lunch			
	Dinner			
	Bedtime			
TUESDAY __/__/__	Breakfast			
	Lunch			
	Dinner			
	Bedtime			
WEDNESDAY __/__/__	Breakfast			
	Lunch			
	Dinner			
	Bedtime			
THURSDAY __/__/__	Breakfast			
	Lunch			
	Dinner			
	Bedtime			
FRIDAY __/__/__	Breakfast			
	Lunch			
	Dinner			
	Bedtime			
SATURDAY __/__/__	Breakfast			
	Lunch			
	Dinner			
	Bedtime			
SUNDAY __/__/__	Breakfast			
	Lunch			
	Dinner			
	Bedtime			

NOTE

Week				Weight

Date	Meal	Before	After	Note
MONDAY __/__/__	Breakfast			
	Lunch			
	Dinner			
	Bedtime			
TUESDAY __/__/__	Breakfast			
	Lunch			
	Dinner			
	Bedtime			
WEDNESDAY __/__/__	Breakfast			
	Lunch			
	Dinner			
	Bedtime			
THURSDAY __/__/__	Breakfast			
	Lunch			
	Dinner			
	Bedtime			
FRIDAY __/__/__	Breakfast			
	Lunch			
	Dinner			
	Bedtime			
SATURDAY __/__/__	Breakfast			
	Lunch			
	Dinner			
	Bedtime			
SUNDAY __/__/__	Breakfast			
	Lunch			
	Dinner			
	Bedtime			

NOTE

Week				Weight

Date	Meal	Before	After	Note
MONDAY __/__/__	Breakfast			
	Lunch			
	Dinner			
	Bedtime			
TUESDAY __/__/__	Breakfast			
	Lunch			
	Dinner			
	Bedtime			
WEDNESDAY __/__/__	Breakfast			
	Lunch			
	Dinner			
	Bedtime			
THURSDAY __/__/__	Breakfast			
	Lunch			
	Dinner			
	Bedtime			
FRIDAY __/__/__	Breakfast			
	Lunch			
	Dinner			
	Bedtime			
SATURDAY __/__/__	Breakfast			
	Lunch			
	Dinner			
	Bedtime			
SUNDAY __/__/__	Breakfast			
	Lunch			
	Dinner			
	Bedtime			

NOTE

Week				Weight

Date	Meal	Before	After	Note
MONDAY ___/___/___	Breakfast			
	Lunch			
	Dinner			
	Bedtime			
TUESDAY ___/___/___	Breakfast			
	Lunch			
	Dinner			
	Bedtime			
WEDNESDAY ___/___/___	Breakfast			
	Lunch			
	Dinner			
	Bedtime			
THURSDAY ___/___/___	Breakfast			
	Lunch			
	Dinner			
	Bedtime			
FRIDAY ___/___/___	Breakfast			
	Lunch			
	Dinner			
	Bedtime			
SATURDAY ___/___/___	Breakfast			
	Lunch			
	Dinner			
	Bedtime			
SUNDAY ___/___/___	Breakfast			
	Lunch			
	Dinner			
	Bedtime			

NOTE

Week				Weight	

Date	Meal	Before	After	Note
MONDAY ___/___/___	Breakfast			
	Lunch			
	Dinner			
	Bedtime			
TUESDAY ___/___/___	Breakfast			
	Lunch			
	Dinner			
	Bedtime			
WEDNESDAY ___/___/___	Breakfast			
	Lunch			
	Dinner			
	Bedtime			
THURSDAY ___/___/___	Breakfast			
	Lunch			
	Dinner			
	Bedtime			
FRIDAY ___/___/___	Breakfast			
	Lunch			
	Dinner			
	Bedtime			
SATURDAY ___/___/___	Breakfast			
	Lunch			
	Dinner			
	Bedtime			
SUNDAY ___/___/___	Breakfast			
	Lunch			
	Dinner			
	Bedtime			

NOTE

Week				Weight

Date	Meal	Before	After	Note
MONDAY __ / __ / __	Breakfast			
	Lunch			
	Dinner			
	Bedtime			
TUESDAY __ / __ / __	Breakfast			
	Lunch			
	Dinner			
	Bedtime			
WEDNESDAY __ / __ / __	Breakfast			
	Lunch			
	Dinner			
	Bedtime			
THURSDAY __ / __ / __	Breakfast			
	Lunch			
	Dinner			
	Bedtime			
FRIDAY __ / __ / __	Breakfast			
	Lunch			
	Dinner			
	Bedtime			
SATURDAY __ / __ / __	Breakfast			
	Lunch			
	Dinner			
	Bedtime			
SUNDAY __ / __ / __	Breakfast			
	Lunch			
	Dinner			
	Bedtime			

NOTE

Week				Weight

Date	Meal	Before	After	Note
MONDAY ___/___/___	Breakfast			
	Lunch			
	Dinner			
	Bedtime			
TUESDAY ___/___/___	Breakfast			
	Lunch			
	Dinner			
	Bedtime			
WEDNESDAY ___/___/___	Breakfast			
	Lunch			
	Dinner			
	Bedtime			
THURSDAY ___/___/___	Breakfast			
	Lunch			
	Dinner			
	Bedtime			
FRIDAY ___/___/___	Breakfast			
	Lunch			
	Dinner			
	Bedtime			
SATURDAY ___/___/___	Breakfast			
	Lunch			
	Dinner			
	Bedtime			
SUNDAY ___/___/___	Breakfast			
	Lunch			
	Dinner			
	Bedtime			

NOTE

Week				Weight

Date	Meal	Before	After	Note
MONDAY ___/___/___	Breakfast			
	Lunch			
	Dinner			
	Bedtime			
TUESDAY ___/___/___	Breakfast			
	Lunch			
	Dinner			
	Bedtime			
WEDNESDAY ___/___/___	Breakfast			
	Lunch			
	Dinner			
	Bedtime			
THURSDAY ___/___/___	Breakfast			
	Lunch			
	Dinner			
	Bedtime			
FRIDAY ___/___/___	Breakfast			
	Lunch			
	Dinner			
	Bedtime			
SATURDAY ___/___/___	Breakfast			
	Lunch			
	Dinner			
	Bedtime			
SUNDAY ___/___/___	Breakfast			
	Lunch			
	Dinner			
	Bedtime			

NOTE

Week				Weight

Date	Meal	Before	After	Note
MONDAY ___/___/___	Breakfast			
	Lunch			
	Dinner			
	Bedtime			
TUESDAY ___/___/___	Breakfast			
	Lunch			
	Dinner			
	Bedtime			
WEDNESDAY ___/___/___	Breakfast			
	Lunch			
	Dinner			
	Bedtime			
THURSDAY ___/___/___	Breakfast			
	Lunch			
	Dinner			
	Bedtime			
FRIDAY ___/___/___	Breakfast			
	Lunch			
	Dinner			
	Bedtime			
SATURDAY ___/___/___	Breakfast			
	Lunch			
	Dinner			
	Bedtime			
SUNDAY ___/___/___	Breakfast			
	Lunch			
	Dinner			
	Bedtime			

NOTE

Week				Weight

Date	Meal	Before	After	Note
MONDAY __/__/__	Breakfast			
	Lunch			
	Dinner			
	Bedtime			
TUESDAY __/__/__	Breakfast			
	Lunch			
	Dinner			
	Bedtime			
WEDNESDAY __/__/__	Breakfast			
	Lunch			
	Dinner			
	Bedtime			
THURSDAY __/__/__	Breakfast			
	Lunch			
	Dinner			
	Bedtime			
FRIDAY __/__/__	Breakfast			
	Lunch			
	Dinner			
	Bedtime			
SATURDAY __/__/__	Breakfast			
	Lunch			
	Dinner			
	Bedtime			
SUNDAY __/__/__	Breakfast			
	Lunch			
	Dinner			
	Bedtime			

NOTE

Week				Weight

Date	Meal	Before	After	Note
MONDAY __/__/__	Breakfast			
	Lunch			
	Dinner			
	Bedtime			
TUESDAY __/__/__	Breakfast			
	Lunch			
	Dinner			
	Bedtime			
WEDNESDAY __/__/__	Breakfast			
	Lunch			
	Dinner			
	Bedtime			
THURSDAY __/__/__	Breakfast			
	Lunch			
	Dinner			
	Bedtime			
FRIDAY __/__/__	Breakfast			
	Lunch			
	Dinner			
	Bedtime			
SATURDAY __/__/__	Breakfast			
	Lunch			
	Dinner			
	Bedtime			
SUNDAY __/__/__	Breakfast			
	Lunch			
	Dinner			
	Bedtime			

NOTE

Week				Weight

Date	Meal	Before	After	Note
MONDAY ___/___/___	Breakfast			
	Lunch			
	Dinner			
	Bedtime			
TUESDAY ___/___/___	Breakfast			
	Lunch			
	Dinner			
	Bedtime			
WEDNESDAY ___/___/___	Breakfast			
	Lunch			
	Dinner			
	Bedtime			
THURSDAY ___/___/___	Breakfast			
	Lunch			
	Dinner			
	Bedtime			
FRIDAY ___/___/___	Breakfast			
	Lunch			
	Dinner			
	Bedtime			
SATURDAY ___/___/___	Breakfast			
	Lunch			
	Dinner			
	Bedtime			
SUNDAY ___/___/___	Breakfast			
	Lunch			
	Dinner			
	Bedtime			

NOTE

Week				Weight

Date	Meal	Before	After	Note
MONDAY __/__/__	Breakfast			
	Lunch			
	Dinner			
	Bedtime			
TUESDAY __/__/__	Breakfast			
	Lunch			
	Dinner			
	Bedtime			
WEDNESDAY __/__/__	Breakfast			
	Lunch			
	Dinner			
	Bedtime			
THURSDAY __/__/__	Breakfast			
	Lunch			
	Dinner			
	Bedtime			
FRIDAY __/__/__	Breakfast			
	Lunch			
	Dinner			
	Bedtime			
SATURDAY __/__/__	Breakfast			
	Lunch			
	Dinner			
	Bedtime			
SUNDAY __/__/__	Breakfast			
	Lunch			
	Dinner			
	Bedtime			

NOTE

Week				Weight

Date	Meal	Before	After	Note
MONDAY __/__/__	Breakfast			
	Lunch			
	Dinner			
	Bedtime			
TUESDAY __/__/__	Breakfast			
	Lunch			
	Dinner			
	Bedtime			
WEDNESDAY __/__/__	Breakfast			
	Lunch			
	Dinner			
	Bedtime			
THURSDAY __/__/__	Breakfast			
	Lunch			
	Dinner			
	Bedtime			
FRIDAY __/__/__	Breakfast			
	Lunch			
	Dinner			
	Bedtime			
SATURDAY __/__/__	Breakfast			
	Lunch			
	Dinner			
	Bedtime			
SUNDAY __/__/__	Breakfast			
	Lunch			
	Dinner			
	Bedtime			

NOTE

Week				Weight

Date	Meal	Before	After	Note
MONDAY __/__/__	Breakfast			
	Lunch			
	Dinner			
	Bedtime			
TUESDAY __/__/__	Breakfast			
	Lunch			
	Dinner			
	Bedtime			
WEDNESDAY __/__/__	Breakfast			
	Lunch			
	Dinner			
	Bedtime			
THURSDAY __/__/__	Breakfast			
	Lunch			
	Dinner			
	Bedtime			
FRIDAY __/__/__	Breakfast			
	Lunch			
	Dinner			
	Bedtime			
SATURDAY __/__/__	Breakfast			
	Lunch			
	Dinner			
	Bedtime			
SUNDAY __/__/__	Breakfast			
	Lunch			
	Dinner			
	Bedtime			

NOTE

Week				Weight

Date	Meal	Before	After	Note
MONDAY ___/___/___	Breakfast			
	Lunch			
	Dinner			
	Bedtime			
TUESDAY ___/___/___	Breakfast			
	Lunch			
	Dinner			
	Bedtime			
WEDNESDAY ___/___/___	Breakfast			
	Lunch			
	Dinner			
	Bedtime			
THURSDAY ___/___/___	Breakfast			
	Lunch			
	Dinner			
	Bedtime			
FRIDAY ___/___/___	Breakfast			
	Lunch			
	Dinner			
	Bedtime			
SATURDAY ___/___/___	Breakfast			
	Lunch			
	Dinner			
	Bedtime			
SUNDAY ___/___/___	Breakfast			
	Lunch			
	Dinner			
	Bedtime			

NOTE

| Week | | | | Weight |

Date	Meal	Before	After	Note
MONDAY ___/___/___	Breakfast			
	Lunch			
	Dinner			
	Bedtime			
TUESDAY ___/___/___	Breakfast			
	Lunch			
	Dinner			
	Bedtime			
WEDNESDAY ___/___/___	Breakfast			
	Lunch			
	Dinner			
	Bedtime			
THURSDAY ___/___/___	Breakfast			
	Lunch			
	Dinner			
	Bedtime			
FRIDAY ___/___/___	Breakfast			
	Lunch			
	Dinner			
	Bedtime			
SATURDAY ___/___/___	Breakfast			
	Lunch			
	Dinner			
	Bedtime			
SUNDAY ___/___/___	Breakfast			
	Lunch			
	Dinner			
	Bedtime			

NOTE

Week				Weight

Date	Meal	Before	After	Note
MONDAY ___/___/___	Breakfast			
	Lunch			
	Dinner			
	Bedtime			
TUESDAY ___/___/___	Breakfast			
	Lunch			
	Dinner			
	Bedtime			
WEDNESDAY ___/___/___	Breakfast			
	Lunch			
	Dinner			
	Bedtime			
THURSDAY ___/___/___	Breakfast			
	Lunch			
	Dinner			
	Bedtime			
FRIDAY ___/___/___	Breakfast			
	Lunch			
	Dinner			
	Bedtime			
SATURDAY ___/___/___	Breakfast			
	Lunch			
	Dinner			
	Bedtime			
SUNDAY ___/___/___	Breakfast			
	Lunch			
	Dinner			
	Bedtime			

NOTE

Week				Weight

Date	Meal	Before	After	Note
MONDAY __/__/__	Breakfast			
	Lunch			
	Dinner			
	Bedtime			
TUESDAY __/__/__	Breakfast			
	Lunch			
	Dinner			
	Bedtime			
WEDNESDAY __/__/__	Breakfast			
	Lunch			
	Dinner			
	Bedtime			
THURSDAY __/__/__	Breakfast			
	Lunch			
	Dinner			
	Bedtime			
FRIDAY __/__/__	Breakfast			
	Lunch			
	Dinner			
	Bedtime			
SATURDAY __/__/__	Breakfast			
	Lunch			
	Dinner			
	Bedtime			
SUNDAY __/__/__	Breakfast			
	Lunch			
	Dinner			
	Bedtime			

NOTE

Week				Weight

Date	Meal	Before	After	Note
MONDAY ___ / ___ / ___	Breakfast			
	Lunch			
	Dinner			
	Bedtime			
TUESDAY ___ / ___ / ___	Breakfast			
	Lunch			
	Dinner			
	Bedtime			
WEDNESDAY ___ / ___ / ___	Breakfast			
	Lunch			
	Dinner			
	Bedtime			
THURSDAY ___ / ___ / ___	Breakfast			
	Lunch			
	Dinner			
	Bedtime			
FRIDAY ___ / ___ / ___	Breakfast			
	Lunch			
	Dinner			
	Bedtime			
SATURDAY ___ / ___ / ___	Breakfast			
	Lunch			
	Dinner			
	Bedtime			
SUNDAY ___ / ___ / ___	Breakfast			
	Lunch			
	Dinner			
	Bedtime			

NOTE

Week				Weight

Date	Meal	Before	After	Note
MONDAY ___/___/___	Breakfast			
	Lunch			
	Dinner			
	Bedtime			
TUESDAY ___/___/___	Breakfast			
	Lunch			
	Dinner			
	Bedtime			
WEDNESDAY ___/___/___	Breakfast			
	Lunch			
	Dinner			
	Bedtime			
THURSDAY ___/___/___	Breakfast			
	Lunch			
	Dinner			
	Bedtime			
FRIDAY ___/___/___	Breakfast			
	Lunch			
	Dinner			
	Bedtime			
SATURDAY ___/___/___	Breakfast			
	Lunch			
	Dinner			
	Bedtime			
SUNDAY ___/___/___	Breakfast			
	Lunch			
	Dinner			
	Bedtime			

NOTE

Week				Weight

Date	Meal	Before	After	Note
MONDAY __/__/__	Breakfast			
	Lunch			
	Dinner			
	Bedtime			
TUESDAY __/__/__	Breakfast			
	Lunch			
	Dinner			
	Bedtime			
WEDNESDAY __/__/__	Breakfast			
	Lunch			
	Dinner			
	Bedtime			
THURSDAY __/__/__	Breakfast			
	Lunch			
	Dinner			
	Bedtime			
FRIDAY __/__/__	Breakfast			
	Lunch			
	Dinner			
	Bedtime			
SATURDAY __/__/__	Breakfast			
	Lunch			
	Dinner			
	Bedtime			
SUNDAY __/__/__	Breakfast			
	Lunch			
	Dinner			
	Bedtime			

NOTE

Week				Weight

Date	Meal	Before	After	Note
MONDAY __/__/__	Breakfast			
	Lunch			
	Dinner			
	Bedtime			
TUESDAY __/__/__	Breakfast			
	Lunch			
	Dinner			
	Bedtime			
WEDNESDAY __/__/__	Breakfast			
	Lunch			
	Dinner			
	Bedtime			
THURSDAY __/__/__	Breakfast			
	Lunch			
	Dinner			
	Bedtime			
FRIDAY __/__/__	Breakfast			
	Lunch			
	Dinner			
	Bedtime			
SATURDAY __/__/__	Breakfast			
	Lunch			
	Dinner			
	Bedtime			
SUNDAY __/__/__	Breakfast			
	Lunch			
	Dinner			
	Bedtime			

NOTE

Week				Weight

Date	Meal	Before	After	Note
MONDAY __/__/__	Breakfast			
	Lunch			
	Dinner			
	Bedtime			
TUESDAY __/__/__	Breakfast			
	Lunch			
	Dinner			
	Bedtime			
WEDNESDAY __/__/__	Breakfast			
	Lunch			
	Dinner			
	Bedtime			
THURSDAY __/__/__	Breakfast			
	Lunch			
	Dinner			
	Bedtime			
FRIDAY __/__/__	Breakfast			
	Lunch			
	Dinner			
	Bedtime			
SATURDAY __/__/__	Breakfast			
	Lunch			
	Dinner			
	Bedtime			
SUNDAY __/__/__	Breakfast			
	Lunch			
	Dinner			
	Bedtime			

NOTE

Week				Weight

Date	Meal	Before	After	Note
MONDAY ___/___/___	Breakfast			
	Lunch			
	Dinner			
	Bedtime			
TUESDAY ___/___/___	Breakfast			
	Lunch			
	Dinner			
	Bedtime			
WEDNESDAY ___/___/___	Breakfast			
	Lunch			
	Dinner			
	Bedtime			
THURSDAY ___/___/___	Breakfast			
	Lunch			
	Dinner			
	Bedtime			
FRIDAY ___/___/___	Breakfast			
	Lunch			
	Dinner			
	Bedtime			
SATURDAY ___/___/___	Breakfast			
	Lunch			
	Dinner			
	Bedtime			
SUNDAY ___/___/___	Breakfast			
	Lunch			
	Dinner			
	Bedtime			

NOTE

Week				Weight

Date	Meal	Before	After	Note
MONDAY ___/___/___	Breakfast			
	Lunch			
	Dinner			
	Bedtime			
TUESDAY ___/___/___	Breakfast			
	Lunch			
	Dinner			
	Bedtime			
WEDNESDAY ___/___/___	Breakfast			
	Lunch			
	Dinner			
	Bedtime			
THURSDAY ___/___/___	Breakfast			
	Lunch			
	Dinner			
	Bedtime			
FRIDAY ___/___/___	Breakfast			
	Lunch			
	Dinner			
	Bedtime			
SATURDAY ___/___/___	Breakfast			
	Lunch			
	Dinner			
	Bedtime			
SUNDAY ___/___/___	Breakfast			
	Lunch			
	Dinner			
	Bedtime			

NOTE

Week				Weight

Date	Meal	Before	After	Note
MONDAY ___/___/___	Breakfast			
	Lunch			
	Dinner			
	Bedtime			
TUESDAY ___/___/___	Breakfast			
	Lunch			
	Dinner			
	Bedtime			
WEDNESDAY ___/___/___	Breakfast			
	Lunch			
	Dinner			
	Bedtime			
THURSDAY ___/___/___	Breakfast			
	Lunch			
	Dinner			
	Bedtime			
FRIDAY ___/___/___	Breakfast			
	Lunch			
	Dinner			
	Bedtime			
SATURDAY ___/___/___	Breakfast			
	Lunch			
	Dinner			
	Bedtime			
SUNDAY ___/___/___	Breakfast			
	Lunch			
	Dinner			
	Bedtime			

NOTE

Week				Weight

Date	Meal	Before	After	Note
MONDAY __/__/__	Breakfast			
	Lunch			
	Dinner			
	Bedtime			
TUESDAY __/__/__	Breakfast			
	Lunch			
	Dinner			
	Bedtime			
WEDNESDAY __/__/__	Breakfast			
	Lunch			
	Dinner			
	Bedtime			
THURSDAY __/__/__	Breakfast			
	Lunch			
	Dinner			
	Bedtime			
FRIDAY __/__/__	Breakfast			
	Lunch			
	Dinner			
	Bedtime			
SATURDAY __/__/__	Breakfast			
	Lunch			
	Dinner			
	Bedtime			
SUNDAY __/__/__	Breakfast			
	Lunch			
	Dinner			
	Bedtime			

NOTE

Week				Weight

Date	Meal	Before	After	Note
MONDAY __/__/__	Breakfast			
	Lunch			
	Dinner			
	Bedtime			
TUESDAY __/__/__	Breakfast			
	Lunch			
	Dinner			
	Bedtime			
WEDNESDAY __/__/__	Breakfast			
	Lunch			
	Dinner			
	Bedtime			
THURSDAY __/__/__	Breakfast			
	Lunch			
	Dinner			
	Bedtime			
FRIDAY __/__/__	Breakfast			
	Lunch			
	Dinner			
	Bedtime			
SATURDAY __/__/__	Breakfast			
	Lunch			
	Dinner			
	Bedtime			
SUNDAY __/__/__	Breakfast			
	Lunch			
	Dinner			
	Bedtime			

NOTE

Week				Weight

Date	Meal	Before	After	Note
MONDAY __/__/__	Breakfast			
	Lunch			
	Dinner			
	Bedtime			
TUESDAY __/__/__	Breakfast			
	Lunch			
	Dinner			
	Bedtime			
WEDNESDAY __/__/__	Breakfast			
	Lunch			
	Dinner			
	Bedtime			
THURSDAY __/__/__	Breakfast			
	Lunch			
	Dinner			
	Bedtime			
FRIDAY __/__/__	Breakfast			
	Lunch			
	Dinner			
	Bedtime			
SATURDAY __/__/__	Breakfast			
	Lunch			
	Dinner			
	Bedtime			
SUNDAY __/__/__	Breakfast			
	Lunch			
	Dinner			
	Bedtime			

NOTE

Week				Weight

Date	Meal	Before	After	Note
MONDAY ___/___/___	Breakfast			
	Lunch			
	Dinner			
	Bedtime			
TUESDAY ___/___/___	Breakfast			
	Lunch			
	Dinner			
	Bedtime			
WEDNESDAY ___/___/___	Breakfast			
	Lunch			
	Dinner			
	Bedtime			
THURSDAY ___/___/___	Breakfast			
	Lunch			
	Dinner			
	Bedtime			
FRIDAY ___/___/___	Breakfast			
	Lunch			
	Dinner			
	Bedtime			
SATURDAY ___/___/___	Breakfast			
	Lunch			
	Dinner			
	Bedtime			
SUNDAY ___/___/___	Breakfast			
	Lunch			
	Dinner			
	Bedtime			

NOTE

Week				Weight

Date	Meal	Before	After	Note
MONDAY ___/___/___	Breakfast			
	Lunch			
	Dinner			
	Bedtime			
TUESDAY ___/___/___	Breakfast			
	Lunch			
	Dinner			
	Bedtime			
WEDNESDAY ___/___/___	Breakfast			
	Lunch			
	Dinner			
	Bedtime			
THURSDAY ___/___/___	Breakfast			
	Lunch			
	Dinner			
	Bedtime			
FRIDAY ___/___/___	Breakfast			
	Lunch			
	Dinner			
	Bedtime			
SATURDAY ___/___/___	Breakfast			
	Lunch			
	Dinner			
	Bedtime			
SUNDAY ___/___/___	Breakfast			
	Lunch			
	Dinner			
	Bedtime			

NOTE

Week				Weight

Date	Meal	Before	After	Note
MONDAY ___/___/___	Breakfast			
	Lunch			
	Dinner			
	Bedtime			
TUESDAY ___/___/___	Breakfast			
	Lunch			
	Dinner			
	Bedtime			
WEDNESDAY ___/___/___	Breakfast			
	Lunch			
	Dinner			
	Bedtime			
THURSDAY ___/___/___	Breakfast			
	Lunch			
	Dinner			
	Bedtime			
FRIDAY ___/___/___	Breakfast			
	Lunch			
	Dinner			
	Bedtime			
SATURDAY ___/___/___	Breakfast			
	Lunch			
	Dinner			
	Bedtime			
SUNDAY ___/___/___	Breakfast			
	Lunch			
	Dinner			
	Bedtime			

NOTE

Week				Weight

Date	Meal	Before	After	Note
MONDAY __ / __ / __	Breakfast			
	Lunch			
	Dinner			
	Bedtime			
TUESDAY __ / __ / __	Breakfast			
	Lunch			
	Dinner			
	Bedtime			
WEDNESDAY __ / __ / __	Breakfast			
	Lunch			
	Dinner			
	Bedtime			
THURSDAY __ / __ / __	Breakfast			
	Lunch			
	Dinner			
	Bedtime			
FRIDAY __ / __ / __	Breakfast			
	Lunch			
	Dinner			
	Bedtime			
SATURDAY __ / __ / __	Breakfast			
	Lunch			
	Dinner			
	Bedtime			
SUNDAY __ / __ / __	Breakfast			
	Lunch			
	Dinner			
	Bedtime			

NOTE

Week				Weight

Date	Meal	Before	After	Note
MONDAY ___/___/___	Breakfast			
	Lunch			
	Dinner			
	Bedtime			
TUESDAY ___/___/___	Breakfast			
	Lunch			
	Dinner			
	Bedtime			
WEDNESDAY ___/___/___	Breakfast			
	Lunch			
	Dinner			
	Bedtime			
THURSDAY ___/___/___	Breakfast			
	Lunch			
	Dinner			
	Bedtime			
FRIDAY ___/___/___	Breakfast			
	Lunch			
	Dinner			
	Bedtime			
SATURDAY ___/___/___	Breakfast			
	Lunch			
	Dinner			
	Bedtime			
SUNDAY ___/___/___	Breakfast			
	Lunch			
	Dinner			
	Bedtime			

NOTE

Week				Weight

Date	Meal	Before	After	Note
MONDAY __/__/__	Breakfast			
	Lunch			
	Dinner			
	Bedtime			
TUESDAY __/__/__	Breakfast			
	Lunch			
	Dinner			
	Bedtime			
WEDNESDAY __/__/__	Breakfast			
	Lunch			
	Dinner			
	Bedtime			
THURSDAY __/__/__	Breakfast			
	Lunch			
	Dinner			
	Bedtime			
FRIDAY __/__/__	Breakfast			
	Lunch			
	Dinner			
	Bedtime			
SATURDAY __/__/__	Breakfast			
	Lunch			
	Dinner			
	Bedtime			
SUNDAY __/__/__	Breakfast			
	Lunch			
	Dinner			
	Bedtime			

NOTE

Week				Weight

Date	Meal	Before	After	Note
MONDAY ___/___/___	Breakfast			
	Lunch			
	Dinner			
	Bedtime			
TUESDAY ___/___/___	Breakfast			
	Lunch			
	Dinner			
	Bedtime			
WEDNESDAY ___/___/___	Breakfast			
	Lunch			
	Dinner			
	Bedtime			
THURSDAY ___/___/___	Breakfast			
	Lunch			
	Dinner			
	Bedtime			
FRIDAY ___/___/___	Breakfast			
	Lunch			
	Dinner			
	Bedtime			
SATURDAY ___/___/___	Breakfast			
	Lunch			
	Dinner			
	Bedtime			
SUNDAY ___/___/___	Breakfast			
	Lunch			
	Dinner			
	Bedtime			

NOTE

Week				Weight

Date	Meal	Before	After	Note
MONDAY __ / __ / __	Breakfast			
	Lunch			
	Dinner			
	Bedtime			
TUESDAY __ / __ / __	Breakfast			
	Lunch			
	Dinner			
	Bedtime			
WEDNESDAY __ / __ / __	Breakfast			
	Lunch			
	Dinner			
	Bedtime			
THURSDAY __ / __ / __	Breakfast			
	Lunch			
	Dinner			
	Bedtime			
FRIDAY __ / __ / __	Breakfast			
	Lunch			
	Dinner			
	Bedtime			
SATURDAY __ / __ / __	Breakfast			
	Lunch			
	Dinner			
	Bedtime			
SUNDAY __ / __ / __	Breakfast			
	Lunch			
	Dinner			
	Bedtime			

NOTE

Week				Weight

Date	Meal	Before	After	Note
MONDAY __/__/__	Breakfast			
	Lunch			
	Dinner			
	Bedtime			
TUESDAY __/__/__	Breakfast			
	Lunch			
	Dinner			
	Bedtime			
WEDNESDAY __/__/__	Breakfast			
	Lunch			
	Dinner			
	Bedtime			
THURSDAY __/__/__	Breakfast			
	Lunch			
	Dinner			
	Bedtime			
FRIDAY __/__/__	Breakfast			
	Lunch			
	Dinner			
	Bedtime			
SATURDAY __/__/__	Breakfast			
	Lunch			
	Dinner			
	Bedtime			
SUNDAY __/__/__	Breakfast			
	Lunch			
	Dinner			
	Bedtime			

NOTE

Week				Weight

Date	Meal	Before	After	Note
MONDAY __/__/__	Breakfast			
	Lunch			
	Dinner			
	Bedtime			
TUESDAY __/__/__	Breakfast			
	Lunch			
	Dinner			
	Bedtime			
WEDNESDAY __/__/__	Breakfast			
	Lunch			
	Dinner			
	Bedtime			
THURSDAY __/__/__	Breakfast			
	Lunch			
	Dinner			
	Bedtime			
FRIDAY __/__/__	Breakfast			
	Lunch			
	Dinner			
	Bedtime			
SATURDAY __/__/__	Breakfast			
	Lunch			
	Dinner			
	Bedtime			
SUNDAY __/__/__	Breakfast			
	Lunch			
	Dinner			
	Bedtime			

NOTE

Week				Weight

Date	Meal	Before	After	Note
MONDAY __/__/__	Breakfast			
	Lunch			
	Dinner			
	Bedtime			
TUESDAY __/__/__	Breakfast			
	Lunch			
	Dinner			
	Bedtime			
WEDNESDAY __/__/__	Breakfast			
	Lunch			
	Dinner			
	Bedtime			
THURSDAY __/__/__	Breakfast			
	Lunch			
	Dinner			
	Bedtime			
FRIDAY __/__/__	Breakfast			
	Lunch			
	Dinner			
	Bedtime			
SATURDAY __/__/__	Breakfast			
	Lunch			
	Dinner			
	Bedtime			
SUNDAY __/__/__	Breakfast			
	Lunch			
	Dinner			
	Bedtime			

NOTE

Week				Weight

Date	Meal	Before	After	Note
MONDAY ___/___/___	Breakfast			
	Lunch			
	Dinner			
	Bedtime			
TUESDAY ___/___/___	Breakfast			
	Lunch			
	Dinner			
	Bedtime			
WEDNESDAY ___/___/___	Breakfast			
	Lunch			
	Dinner			
	Bedtime			
THURSDAY ___/___/___	Breakfast			
	Lunch			
	Dinner			
	Bedtime			
FRIDAY ___/___/___	Breakfast			
	Lunch			
	Dinner			
	Bedtime			
SATURDAY ___/___/___	Breakfast			
	Lunch			
	Dinner			
	Bedtime			
SUNDAY ___/___/___	Breakfast			
	Lunch			
	Dinner			
	Bedtime			

NOTE

Week				Weight

Date	Meal	Before	After	Note
MONDAY ___/___/___	Breakfast			
	Lunch			
	Dinner			
	Bedtime			
TUESDAY ___/___/___	Breakfast			
	Lunch			
	Dinner			
	Bedtime			
WEDNESDAY ___/___/___	Breakfast			
	Lunch			
	Dinner			
	Bedtime			
THURSDAY ___/___/___	Breakfast			
	Lunch			
	Dinner			
	Bedtime			
FRIDAY ___/___/___	Breakfast			
	Lunch			
	Dinner			
	Bedtime			
SATURDAY ___/___/___	Breakfast			
	Lunch			
	Dinner			
	Bedtime			
SUNDAY ___/___/___	Breakfast			
	Lunch			
	Dinner			
	Bedtime			

NOTE

Week				Weight

Date	Meal	Before	After	Note
MONDAY __/__/__	Breakfast			
	Lunch			
	Dinner			
	Bedtime			
TUESDAY __/__/__	Breakfast			
	Lunch			
	Dinner			
	Bedtime			
WEDNESDAY __/__/__	Breakfast			
	Lunch			
	Dinner			
	Bedtime			
THURSDAY __/__/__	Breakfast			
	Lunch			
	Dinner			
	Bedtime			
FRIDAY __/__/__	Breakfast			
	Lunch			
	Dinner			
	Bedtime			
SATURDAY __/__/__	Breakfast			
	Lunch			
	Dinner			
	Bedtime			
SUNDAY __/__/__	Breakfast			
	Lunch			
	Dinner			
	Bedtime			

NOTE

Week				Weight

Date	Meal	Before	After	Note
MONDAY __/__/__	Breakfast			
	Lunch			
	Dinner			
	Bedtime			
TUESDAY __/__/__	Breakfast			
	Lunch			
	Dinner			
	Bedtime			
WEDNESDAY __/__/__	Breakfast			
	Lunch			
	Dinner			
	Bedtime			
THURSDAY __/__/__	Breakfast			
	Lunch			
	Dinner			
	Bedtime			
FRIDAY __/__/__	Breakfast			
	Lunch			
	Dinner			
	Bedtime			
SATURDAY __/__/__	Breakfast			
	Lunch			
	Dinner			
	Bedtime			
SUNDAY __/__/__	Breakfast			
	Lunch			
	Dinner			
	Bedtime			

NOTE

Week				Weight

Date	Meal	Before	After	Note
MONDAY __/__/__	Breakfast			
	Lunch			
	Dinner			
	Bedtime			
TUESDAY __/__/__	Breakfast			
	Lunch			
	Dinner			
	Bedtime			
WEDNESDAY __/__/__	Breakfast			
	Lunch			
	Dinner			
	Bedtime			
THURSDAY __/__/__	Breakfast			
	Lunch			
	Dinner			
	Bedtime			
FRIDAY __/__/__	Breakfast			
	Lunch			
	Dinner			
	Bedtime			
SATURDAY __/__/__	Breakfast			
	Lunch			
	Dinner			
	Bedtime			
SUNDAY __/__/__	Breakfast			
	Lunch			
	Dinner			
	Bedtime			

NOTE

Week				Weight

Date	Meal	Before	After	Note
MONDAY ___/___/___	Breakfast			
	Lunch			
	Dinner			
	Bedtime			
TUESDAY ___/___/___	Breakfast			
	Lunch			
	Dinner			
	Bedtime			
WEDNESDAY ___/___/___	Breakfast			
	Lunch			
	Dinner			
	Bedtime			
THURSDAY ___/___/___	Breakfast			
	Lunch			
	Dinner			
	Bedtime			
FRIDAY ___/___/___	Breakfast			
	Lunch			
	Dinner			
	Bedtime			
SATURDAY ___/___/___	Breakfast			
	Lunch			
	Dinner			
	Bedtime			
SUNDAY ___/___/___	Breakfast			
	Lunch			
	Dinner			
	Bedtime			

NOTE

Week				Weight

Date	Meal	Before	After	Note
MONDAY ___/___/___	Breakfast			
	Lunch			
	Dinner			
	Bedtime			
TUESDAY ___/___/___	Breakfast			
	Lunch			
	Dinner			
	Bedtime			
WEDNESDAY ___/___/___	Breakfast			
	Lunch			
	Dinner			
	Bedtime			
THURSDAY ___/___/___	Breakfast			
	Lunch			
	Dinner			
	Bedtime			
FRIDAY ___/___/___	Breakfast			
	Lunch			
	Dinner			
	Bedtime			
SATURDAY ___/___/___	Breakfast			
	Lunch			
	Dinner			
	Bedtime			
SUNDAY ___/___/___	Breakfast			
	Lunch			
	Dinner			
	Bedtime			

NOTE

Week				Weight

Date	Meal	Before	After	Note
MONDAY __/__/__	Breakfast			
	Lunch			
	Dinner			
	Bedtime			
TUESDAY __/__/__	Breakfast			
	Lunch			
	Dinner			
	Bedtime			
WEDNESDAY __/__/__	Breakfast			
	Lunch			
	Dinner			
	Bedtime			
THURSDAY __/__/__	Breakfast			
	Lunch			
	Dinner			
	Bedtime			
FRIDAY __/__/__	Breakfast			
	Lunch			
	Dinner			
	Bedtime			
SATURDAY __/__/__	Breakfast			
	Lunch			
	Dinner			
	Bedtime			
SUNDAY __/__/__	Breakfast			
	Lunch			
	Dinner			
	Bedtime			

NOTE

Week				Weight

Date	Meal	Before	After	Note
MONDAY ___ / ___ / ___	Breakfast			
	Lunch			
	Dinner			
	Bedtime			
TUESDAY ___ / ___ / ___	Breakfast			
	Lunch			
	Dinner			
	Bedtime			
WEDNESDAY ___ / ___ / ___	Breakfast			
	Lunch			
	Dinner			
	Bedtime			
THURSDAY ___ / ___ / ___	Breakfast			
	Lunch			
	Dinner			
	Bedtime			
FRIDAY ___ / ___ / ___	Breakfast			
	Lunch			
	Dinner			
	Bedtime			
SATURDAY ___ / ___ / ___	Breakfast			
	Lunch			
	Dinner			
	Bedtime			
SUNDAY ___ / ___ / ___	Breakfast			
	Lunch			
	Dinner			
	Bedtime			

NOTE

Week				Weight

Date	Meal	Before	After	Note
MONDAY ___/___/___	Breakfast			
	Lunch			
	Dinner			
	Bedtime			
TUESDAY ___/___/___	Breakfast			
	Lunch			
	Dinner			
	Bedtime			
WEDNESDAY ___/___/___	Breakfast			
	Lunch			
	Dinner			
	Bedtime			
THURSDAY ___/___/___	Breakfast			
	Lunch			
	Dinner			
	Bedtime			
FRIDAY ___/___/___	Breakfast			
	Lunch			
	Dinner			
	Bedtime			
SATURDAY ___/___/___	Breakfast			
	Lunch			
	Dinner			
	Bedtime			
SUNDAY ___/___/___	Breakfast			
	Lunch			
	Dinner			
	Bedtime			

NOTE _____

_____

Week				Weight

Date	Meal	Before	After	Note
MONDAY ___/___/___	Breakfast			
	Lunch			
	Dinner			
	Bedtime			
TUESDAY ___/___/___	Breakfast			
	Lunch			
	Dinner			
	Bedtime			
WEDNESDAY ___/___/___	Breakfast			
	Lunch			
	Dinner			
	Bedtime			
THURSDAY ___/___/___	Breakfast			
	Lunch			
	Dinner			
	Bedtime			
FRIDAY ___/___/___	Breakfast			
	Lunch			
	Dinner			
	Bedtime			
SATURDAY ___/___/___	Breakfast			
	Lunch			
	Dinner			
	Bedtime			
SUNDAY ___/___/___	Breakfast			
	Lunch			
	Dinner			
	Bedtime			

NOTE

Week				Weight

Date	Meal	Before	After	Note
MONDAY __/__/__	Breakfast			
	Lunch			
	Dinner			
	Bedtime			
TUESDAY __/__/__	Breakfast			
	Lunch			
	Dinner			
	Bedtime			
WEDNESDAY __/__/__	Breakfast			
	Lunch			
	Dinner			
	Bedtime			
THURSDAY __/__/__	Breakfast			
	Lunch			
	Dinner			
	Bedtime			
FRIDAY __/__/__	Breakfast			
	Lunch			
	Dinner			
	Bedtime			
SATURDAY __/__/__	Breakfast			
	Lunch			
	Dinner			
	Bedtime			
SUNDAY __/__/__	Breakfast			
	Lunch			
	Dinner			
	Bedtime			

NOTE

Week				Weight

Date	Meal	Before	After	Note
MONDAY __/__/__	Breakfast			
	Lunch			
	Dinner			
	Bedtime			
TUESDAY __/__/__	Breakfast			
	Lunch			
	Dinner			
	Bedtime			
WEDNESDAY __/__/__	Breakfast			
	Lunch			
	Dinner			
	Bedtime			
THURSDAY __/__/__	Breakfast			
	Lunch			
	Dinner			
	Bedtime			
FRIDAY __/__/__	Breakfast			
	Lunch			
	Dinner			
	Bedtime			
SATURDAY __/__/__	Breakfast			
	Lunch			
	Dinner			
	Bedtime			
SUNDAY __/__/__	Breakfast			
	Lunch			
	Dinner			
	Bedtime			

NOTE

Week				Weight

Date	Meal	Before	After	Note
MONDAY ___/___/___	Breakfast			
	Lunch			
	Dinner			
	Bedtime			
TUESDAY ___/___/___	Breakfast			
	Lunch			
	Dinner			
	Bedtime			
WEDNESDAY ___/___/___	Breakfast			
	Lunch			
	Dinner			
	Bedtime			
THURSDAY ___/___/___	Breakfast			
	Lunch			
	Dinner			
	Bedtime			
FRIDAY ___/___/___	Breakfast			
	Lunch			
	Dinner			
	Bedtime			
SATURDAY ___/___/___	Breakfast			
	Lunch			
	Dinner			
	Bedtime			
SUNDAY ___/___/___	Breakfast			
	Lunch			
	Dinner			
	Bedtime			

NOTE

Week				Weight

Date	Meal	Before	After	Note
MONDAY ___/___/___	Breakfast			
	Lunch			
	Dinner			
	Bedtime			
TUESDAY ___/___/___	Breakfast			
	Lunch			
	Dinner			
	Bedtime			
WEDNESDAY ___/___/___	Breakfast			
	Lunch			
	Dinner			
	Bedtime			
THURSDAY ___/___/___	Breakfast			
	Lunch			
	Dinner			
	Bedtime			
FRIDAY ___/___/___	Breakfast			
	Lunch			
	Dinner			
	Bedtime			
SATURDAY ___/___/___	Breakfast			
	Lunch			
	Dinner			
	Bedtime			
SUNDAY ___/___/___	Breakfast			
	Lunch			
	Dinner			
	Bedtime			

NOTE

Week				Weight

Date	Meal	Before	After	Note
MONDAY __/__/__	Breakfast			
	Lunch			
	Dinner			
	Bedtime			
TUESDAY __/__/__	Breakfast			
	Lunch			
	Dinner			
	Bedtime			
WEDNESDAY __/__/__	Breakfast			
	Lunch			
	Dinner			
	Bedtime			
THURSDAY __/__/__	Breakfast			
	Lunch			
	Dinner			
	Bedtime			
FRIDAY __/__/__	Breakfast			
	Lunch			
	Dinner			
	Bedtime			
SATURDAY __/__/__	Breakfast			
	Lunch			
	Dinner			
	Bedtime			
SUNDAY __/__/__	Breakfast			
	Lunch			
	Dinner			
	Bedtime			

NOTE

Week				Weight

Date	Meal	Before	After	Note
MONDAY __/__/__	Breakfast			
	Lunch			
	Dinner			
	Bedtime			
TUESDAY __/__/__	Breakfast			
	Lunch			
	Dinner			
	Bedtime			
WEDNESDAY __/__/__	Breakfast			
	Lunch			
	Dinner			
	Bedtime			
THURSDAY __/__/__	Breakfast			
	Lunch			
	Dinner			
	Bedtime			
FRIDAY __/__/__	Breakfast			
	Lunch			
	Dinner			
	Bedtime			
SATURDAY __/__/__	Breakfast			
	Lunch			
	Dinner			
	Bedtime			
SUNDAY __/__/__	Breakfast			
	Lunch			
	Dinner			
	Bedtime			

NOTE

Week				Weight

Date	Meal	Before	After	Note
MONDAY __/__/__	Breakfast			
	Lunch			
	Dinner			
	Bedtime			
TUESDAY __/__/__	Breakfast			
	Lunch			
	Dinner			
	Bedtime			
WEDNESDAY __/__/__	Breakfast			
	Lunch			
	Dinner			
	Bedtime			
THURSDAY __/__/__	Breakfast			
	Lunch			
	Dinner			
	Bedtime			
FRIDAY __/__/__	Breakfast			
	Lunch			
	Dinner			
	Bedtime			
SATURDAY __/__/__	Breakfast			
	Lunch			
	Dinner			
	Bedtime			
SUNDAY __/__/__	Breakfast			
	Lunch			
	Dinner			
	Bedtime			

NOTE

Week				Weight

Date	Meal	Before	After	Note
MONDAY ___/___/___	Breakfast			
	Lunch			
	Dinner			
	Bedtime			
TUESDAY ___/___/___	Breakfast			
	Lunch			
	Dinner			
	Bedtime			
WEDNESDAY ___/___/___	Breakfast			
	Lunch			
	Dinner			
	Bedtime			
THURSDAY ___/___/___	Breakfast			
	Lunch			
	Dinner			
	Bedtime			
FRIDAY ___/___/___	Breakfast			
	Lunch			
	Dinner			
	Bedtime			
SATURDAY ___/___/___	Breakfast			
	Lunch			
	Dinner			
	Bedtime			
SUNDAY ___/___/___	Breakfast			
	Lunch			
	Dinner			
	Bedtime			

NOTE

Week				Weight

Date	Meal	Before	After	Note
MONDAY ___/___/___	Breakfast			
	Lunch			
	Dinner			
	Bedtime			
TUESDAY ___/___/___	Breakfast			
	Lunch			
	Dinner			
	Bedtime			
WEDNESDAY ___/___/___	Breakfast			
	Lunch			
	Dinner			
	Bedtime			
THURSDAY ___/___/___	Breakfast			
	Lunch			
	Dinner			
	Bedtime			
FRIDAY ___/___/___	Breakfast			
	Lunch			
	Dinner			
	Bedtime			
SATURDAY ___/___/___	Breakfast			
	Lunch			
	Dinner			
	Bedtime			
SUNDAY ___/___/___	Breakfast			
	Lunch			
	Dinner			
	Bedtime			

NOTE

Week				Weight

Date	Meal	Before	After	Note
MONDAY ___/___/___	Breakfast			
	Lunch			
	Dinner			
	Bedtime			
TUESDAY ___/___/___	Breakfast			
	Lunch			
	Dinner			
	Bedtime			
WEDNESDAY ___/___/___	Breakfast			
	Lunch			
	Dinner			
	Bedtime			
THURSDAY ___/___/___	Breakfast			
	Lunch			
	Dinner			
	Bedtime			
FRIDAY ___/___/___	Breakfast			
	Lunch			
	Dinner			
	Bedtime			
SATURDAY ___/___/___	Breakfast			
	Lunch			
	Dinner			
	Bedtime			
SUNDAY ___/___/___	Breakfast			
	Lunch			
	Dinner			
	Bedtime			

NOTE

Week				Weight

Date	Meal	Before	After	Note
MONDAY __/__/__	Breakfast			
	Lunch			
	Dinner			
	Bedtime			
TUESDAY __/__/__	Breakfast			
	Lunch			
	Dinner			
	Bedtime			
WEDNESDAY __/__/__	Breakfast			
	Lunch			
	Dinner			
	Bedtime			
THURSDAY __/__/__	Breakfast			
	Lunch			
	Dinner			
	Bedtime			
FRIDAY __/__/__	Breakfast			
	Lunch			
	Dinner			
	Bedtime			
SATURDAY __/__/__	Breakfast			
	Lunch			
	Dinner			
	Bedtime			
SUNDAY __/__/__	Breakfast			
	Lunch			
	Dinner			
	Bedtime			

NOTE

Week				Weight

Date	Meal	Before	After	Note
MONDAY ___/___/___	Breakfast			
	Lunch			
	Dinner			
	Bedtime			
TUESDAY ___/___/___	Breakfast			
	Lunch			
	Dinner			
	Bedtime			
WEDNESDAY ___/___/___	Breakfast			
	Lunch			
	Dinner			
	Bedtime			
THURSDAY ___/___/___	Breakfast			
	Lunch			
	Dinner			
	Bedtime			
FRIDAY ___/___/___	Breakfast			
	Lunch			
	Dinner			
	Bedtime			
SATURDAY ___/___/___	Breakfast			
	Lunch			
	Dinner			
	Bedtime			
SUNDAY ___/___/___	Breakfast			
	Lunch			
	Dinner			
	Bedtime			

NOTE

Week				Weight

Date	Meal	Before	After	Note
MONDAY ___/___/___	Breakfast			
	Lunch			
	Dinner			
	Bedtime			
TUESDAY ___/___/___	Breakfast			
	Lunch			
	Dinner			
	Bedtime			
WEDNESDAY ___/___/___	Breakfast			
	Lunch			
	Dinner			
	Bedtime			
THURSDAY ___/___/___	Breakfast			
	Lunch			
	Dinner			
	Bedtime			
FRIDAY ___/___/___	Breakfast			
	Lunch			
	Dinner			
	Bedtime			
SATURDAY ___/___/___	Breakfast			
	Lunch			
	Dinner			
	Bedtime			
SUNDAY ___/___/___	Breakfast			
	Lunch			
	Dinner			
	Bedtime			

NOTE

Made in the USA
Monee, IL
26 November 2024

71330944R00066